"10 minutes of seated workouts for mature individuals":

Quick and effective exercise to keep you active and energized even when sitting down!!!

BY

Dorothy Cooke

TABLE OF CONTENT

Introduction

The Importance of Staying Active

As we age, staying physically active becomes increasingly important for maintaining overall health, well-being, and quality of life. Physical activity helps to manage weight, improve cardiovascular health, enhance muscle strength, and boost mental health. However, as we grow older, it can become more challenging to engage in traditional forms of exercise due to mobility issues, chronic pain, or other health conditions. This is where the concept of seated workouts comes into play.

Physical Health Benefits

- **Cardiovascular Health**: Regular physical activity, even in a seated position, can help maintain heart health by improving circulation, lowering blood pressure, and reducing the risk of heart disease. Engaging in exercises that raise the heart rate, such as seated marching or arm punches, can provide cardiovascular benefits like those of more intense activities.

- **Strength and Endurance**: As we age, muscle mass and strength naturally decline. Seated workouts can help counteract this by providing resistance exercises that build and maintain muscle strength. Exercises like seated leg lifts, bicep curls, and triceps extensions help to keep muscles toned and functional, which is essential for daily activities.

- **Flexibility and Balance**: Flexibility decreases with age, which can lead to stiffness and a higher risk of injuries. Seated stretches, such as neck stretches, seated forward bends, and ankle rotations, help maintain and improve flexibility. Additionally, exercises that focus on core strength and stability, like seated torso twists and pelvic tilts, can enhance balance and reduce the risk of falls.

- **Bone Health**: Weight-bearing workouts have been shown to strengthen bones and lower the incidence of osteoporosis. While seated exercises are not weight-bearing in the traditional sense, they still provide some resistance that can be beneficial for bone health. Additionally, exercises that promote joint movement, like seated rowing and shoulder shrugs, can help maintain joint health and mobility.

- **Chronic Disease Management**: For those living with chronic conditions such as arthritis, diabetes, or hypertension, regular physical activity can help manage symptoms and improve overall health. Seated workouts are a low-impact way to stay active without exacerbating pain or discomfort associated with these conditions. Exercise can help control blood sugar levels, improve joint function, and enhance overall energy levels.

Mental and Emotional Benefits

- **Mood Enhancement**: Physical activity triggers the release of endorphins, which are chemicals in the brain that promote feelings of happiness and well-being. Regular exercise can help combat feelings of depression and anxiety, providing a natural mood boost.

- Cognitive Function: Exercise has been demonstrated to boost cognitive function and lower the risk of cognitive decline. Activities that require coordination and concentration, such as seated tap dance or complex arm movements, can stimulate brain activity and enhance cognitive abilities.
- **Stress Reduction**: Engaging in physical activity can reduce levels of the body's stress hormones, such as adrenaline and cortisol. It also boosts the creation of endorphins, which work as natural pain relievers and mood boosters. This can lead to improved stress management and a greater sense of calm and relaxation.
- **Social Interaction**: Group exercise classes, even those conducted virtually, can provide a sense of community and social interaction. This can assist in alleviating emotions of loneliness and isolation, which are frequent among older people.

Functional Benefits

- **Independence**: Maintaining physical strength and mobility through regular exercise can help older adults remain independent for longer. This means being able to perform daily tasks, such as getting up from a chair, walking, and carrying groceries, with greater ease and less assistance.
- **Quality of Life**: Regular physical activity can enhance overall quality of life by improving physical health, boosting mood, and providing opportunities for social interaction. This can lead to a greater sense of well-being and satisfaction with life.

Benefits of Seated Workouts

Seated workouts offer a unique and effective way to stay active, especially for those who may have difficulty standing or moving for extended periods. These exercises can be adapted to various fitness levels and health conditions, making them accessible to a wide range of individuals.

- **Adaptable for Different Fitness Levels**: Seated workouts can be easily modified to suit different fitness levels. Beginners can start with basic movements, while more advanced individuals can increase the intensity or add resistance bands and light weights to their exercises.
- **Suitable for Various Health Conditions**: For those with chronic pain, joint issues, or mobility limitations, seated exercises provide a low-impact alternative to traditional workouts. This makes it easier to stay active without causing additional strain or discomfort.
- **Convenience**: Seated workouts can be performed almost anywhere, whether at home, in a community center, or even at work. All that is needed is a sturdy chair, making it a convenient option for incorporating physical activity into daily routines.

Comprehensive Workouts

- **Full-Body Engagement**: Seated workouts can be designed to engage all major muscle groups, providing a comprehensive full-body workout. This includes exercises for the upper body, lower body, and core, ensuring balanced muscle development and overall fitness.
- **Combination of Cardio, Strength, and Flexibility**: Seated workouts can incorporate elements of cardiovascular exercise, strength training, and flexibility exercises. This combination helps to improve heart health, build muscle, and enhance flexibility, all from a seated position.

Mental and Emotional Well-Being

- **Increased Confidence**: Regularly participating in seated workouts can boost confidence and self-esteem by providing a sense of accomplishment and progress. Knowing that you are taking steps to improve your health can lead to a more positive outlook on life.

- **Routine and Structure**: Incorporating seated workouts into your daily routine can provide a sense of structure and purpose. This can be particularly beneficial for those who may feel aimless or unmotivated.

Safety and Comfort

- **Reduced Risk of Injury**: Seated exercises reduce the risk of falls and injuries, which can be a concern for older adults. By performing exercises while seated, individuals can focus on their movements without worrying about balance or stability.
- **Comfort and Support**: Sitting in a chair provides support and comfort, allowing individuals to perform exercises without straining their bodies. This is particularly beneficial for those with back pain, arthritis, or other conditions that make standing or lying down uncomfortable.

Longevity and Sustainability

- **Sustainable Exercise Routine**: Seated workouts offer a sustainable way to stay active over the long term. As they can be easily adapted and performed without the need for specialized equipment, they are a practical option for maintaining physical activity throughout life.
- **Consistency**: The ease and convenience of seated workouts make it more likely that individuals will stick with their exercise routine. Consistency is key to reaping the long-term benefits of physical activity, and seated workouts provide a manageable way to stay consistent.

Conclusion

Staying active is crucial for maintaining physical health, mental well-being, and overall quality of life, especially as we age. Seated workouts offer an accessible, effective, and sustainable way for mature individuals to stay active, regardless of their fitness level or health condition. By incorporating seated exercises into your daily routine, you can enjoy the numerous benefits of physical activity while ensuring safety, comfort, and inclusivity.

This book will guide you through various seated workouts, helping you stay active, energized, and engaged, even while sitting down.

Chapter 1: Getting Started

Embarking on a fitness journey with seated workouts is an excellent decision, especially for mature individuals. This chapter provides essential guidelines to help you prepare for your exercise routines, ensuring that you have the right environment, equipment, and knowledge to stay safe and effective. We will cover the following key areas: preparing your space, necessary equipment, safety tips, and warm-up techniques.

a. Preparing Your Space

Creating a dedicated exercise area is crucial for both safety and motivation. Here's how to set up your space for seated workouts:

1. Choose the Right Location:

- **Quiet and Private:** Select a spot in your home that is quiet and free from distractions. This could be a corner of your living room, a spare bedroom, or even a section of your office.
- **Well-Lit:** Ensure the area is well-lit to prevent any accidents and to create a pleasant environment for your workouts.

2. Ensure Adequate Space:

- **Clear Area:** Clear enough space around your chair so you can move your arms and legs freely without knocking into furniture or other objects. Aim for at least three feet of clearance on all sides of the chair.

- **Stability:** Choose a flat, non-slip surface for your workout area. If you're on a hard floor, consider placing a non-slip mat under your chair to prevent it from sliding.

3. Comfortable Environment:

- **Temperature:** Ensure the room temperature is comfortable, neither too hot nor too cold. Exercising in extreme temperatures can be uncomfortable and potentially harmful.
- **Ventilation:** Good ventilation is essential. If possible, exercise in a room with windows that can be opened for fresh air.

b. Necessary Equipment

While seated workouts require minimal equipment, having the right tools can enhance your exercise experience and effectiveness. Here's a list of necessary and optional equipment:

1. Essential Equipment:

- **Sturdy Chair:** The most crucial piece of equipment is a sturdy chair with a straight back. Avoid chairs with wheels or those that recline. A dining chair or an office chair without armrests is ideal.
- **Comfortable Clothing:** Wear comfortable, non-restrictive clothing that allows you to move freely. Avoid tight clothing that can limit your range of motion or cause discomfort.

2. Optional Equipment:

- **Resistance Bands:** These are great for adding resistance to your workouts and can help build strength. Choose bands with different resistance levels to vary the intensity of your exercises.
- **Light Dumbbells:** Light weights (1-3 pounds) can enhance strength training exercises. If you don't have dumbbells, you can use household items like water bottles or canned goods.
- **Exercise Mat:** If you plan to do floor exercises in addition to seated ones, an exercise mat can provide comfort and support.
- **Water Bottle:** Staying hydrated is essential, so keep a water bottle nearby to drink during your workouts.

- **Towel:** A small towel can be handy for wiping away sweat and for certain stretching exercises.

c. Safety Tips

Safety is paramount when engaging in any form of exercise, especially for mature individuals. Here are some safety tips to keep in mind:

1. Consult Your Doctor:

- **Medical Clearance:** Before starting any new exercise program, especially if you have pre-existing health conditions, consult your healthcare provider. They may offer individualized coaching and guarantee that the workouts are safe for you.

2. Start Slow:

- **Gradual Progression:** Begin with basic exercises and gradually increase the intensity and duration as your fitness improves. Pushing oneself too hard too soon might result in an injury.

3. Listen to Your Body:

- **Pain vs. Discomfort:** It's normal to feel some discomfort when you start exercising, but you should never feel pain. If you experience sharp or severe pain, stop the exercise immediately and consult a healthcare professional.
- **Rest When Needed:** Allow yourself to rest if you feel fatigued or dizzy. It's better to take breaks than to overexert yourself.

4. Maintain Proper Form:

- **Correct Technique:** Focus on performing each exercise with proper form. This reduces the risk of injury and ensures you get the most benefit from the exercise. If you're unsure about your form, consider seeking guidance from a fitness professional.

5. Stay Hydrated:

- **Regular Hydration:** Drink water before, during, and after your workout to stay hydrated. Dehydration can lead to dizziness and muscle cramps.

6. Use Supportive Footwear:

- **Proper Shoes:** Wear supportive, non-slip shoes to provide stability and reduce the risk of slipping, especially if you're doing exercises that involve standing or moving from the seated position.

d. Warm-Up Techniques

Warming up is an essential part of any exercise routine. It prepares your body for physical activity by gradually increasing your heart rate, improving blood flow to your muscles, and reducing the risk of injury. Here are some effective warm-up techniques for seated workouts:

1. Seated Marching:

- **How to Do It:** Sit up straight and place your feet flat on the floor. Lift your right knee to your chest, then lower it back down. Repeat with your left knee. Continue alternating legs in a marching motion.
- **Duration:** 1-2 minutes
- **Benefits:** This exercise warms up your leg muscles and gets your heart rate up.

2. Shoulder Rolls:

- **How to Do It:** Sit with your back straight and your feet flat on the floor. Lift your shoulders to your ears, then roll them back and forth in a circular motion. Repeat many times before reversing the direction.
- **Duration:** 1-2 minutes
- **Benefits:** Shoulder rolls loosen up the muscles around your shoulders and upper back, improving flexibility and reducing tension.

3. Arm Circles:

- **How to Do It:** Extend your arms to the sides, shoulder height. Make little circles with your arms and progressively increase the size of the circles. After 10-15 seconds, reverse the direction.
- **Duration:** 1-2 minutes
- **Benefits:** Arm circles warm up your shoulder joints and arm muscles, preparing them for more strenuous activities.

4. Neck Stretches:

- **How to Do It:** Sit up straight with your feet flat on the floor. Gently tilt your head towards your right shoulder, feeling a stretch along the left side of your neck. Hold for 10-15 seconds, then switch sides. Repeat a few times on each side.
- **Duration:** 1-2 minutes
- **Benefits:** Neck stretches help to reduce stiffness and tension in the neck, improving flexibility and preventing strain.

5. Ankle Rotations:

- **How to Do It:** Sit up straight and lift one foot off the floor. Rotate your ankle in a circular motion, first in one direction, then the other. Repeat with the other ankle.
- **Duration:** 1-2 minutes
- **Benefits:** Ankle rotations warm up the muscles and joints in your feet and ankles, enhancing mobility and reducing the risk of injury.

6. Torso Twists:

- **How to Do It:** Sit with your feet flat on the floor and your back straight. Put your hands on your hips or across your chest. Gently twist your torso to the right, then return to the center and twist to the left. Continue alternating sides.
- **Duration:** 1-2 minutes
- **Benefits:** Torso twists warm up the muscles in your core and lower back, improving flexibility and range of motion.

Conclusion

By taking the time to prepare your space, gather the necessary equipment, and follow safety tips, you can set yourself up for success with your seated workouts. Warming up properly ensures that your body is ready for exercise, reducing the risk of injury and enhancing your performance. With these foundations in place, you're ready to embark on your fitness journey and enjoy the numerous benefits of staying active, even from a seated position.

Chapter 2: Upper Body Workouts

Upper body strength is crucial for daily activities and maintaining independence, especially as we age. This chapter focuses on exercises that target the arms, shoulders, and upper back, all of which can be performed while seated. Here's a detailed guide to some effective upper body workouts: Arm Circles and Shoulder Shrugs, Overhead Arm Lifts, Bicep Curls with a Resistance Band, and Triceps Dips using a Chair.

Arm Circles

Arm circles are a simple yet effective exercise that targets the shoulders, upper arms, and upper back. They are excellent for improving flexibility, increasing blood flow to the upper body, and warming up before more strenuous activities.

How to Do Arm Circles:

- **Starting Position:** Sit up straight in a sturdy chair with your feet flat on the floor and your back away from the chair's backrest. Extend your arms out to the sides at shoulder height, keeping them parallel to the floor.
- **Small Circles:** Begin by making small circles with your arms, moving them forward. Keep your movements controlled and your arms straight. Continue for about 30 seconds.
- **Increase Circle Size:** Gradually increase the size of the circles over the next 30 seconds. Ensure that your shoulders are engaged, and your movements are smooth.
- **Reverse Direction:** After one minute, reverse the direction of the circles, starting small and gradually increasing the size. Continue for another minute.

Tips for Arm Circles:

- Maintain a neutral spine and avoid arching your back.
- Keep your movements controlled to maximize the effectiveness and minimize the risk of injury.
- If you experience any discomfort, reduce the size of the circles or take a break.

Shoulder Shrugs

Shoulder shrugs are an excellent exercise for relieving tension and strengthening the muscles around the neck and upper shoulders. This exercise can help improve posture and reduce the risk of shoulder and neck pain.

How to Do Shoulder Shrugs:

- **Starting Position:** Sit up straight with your feet flat on the floor and your hands resting on your thighs or hanging by your sides.
- **Lift Shoulders:** Slowly lift your shoulders towards your ears as if trying to touch them. Hold the lifted position for a few seconds, feeling the muscles contract.
- **Lower Shoulders:** Gradually lower your shoulders back to the starting position, allowing them to relax completely.
- **Repeat:** Perform 10-15 repetitions, focusing on controlled movements.

Tips for Shoulder Shrugs:

- Avoid rolling your shoulders; the movement should be directly up and down.
- Keep your neck relaxed and avoid tensing your jaw.
- Perform the exercise slowly to maximize the contraction and relaxation of the muscles.

b. Overhead Arm Lifts

Overhead arm lifts target the shoulders, upper back, and triceps. This exercise helps to improve shoulder mobility, strengthen the upper body, and enhance overall flexibility.

How to Do Overhead Arm Lifts:

- **Starting Position:** Sit up straight with your feet flat on the floor and your back away from the chair's backrest. Hold a light weight (or a water bottle) in each hand with your arms resting at your sides.
- **Lift Arms:** Slowly lift both arms overhead, keeping them straight. Ensure that your palms are facing each other as your arms rise.
- **Full Extension:** Extend your arms fully above your head without locking your elbows. Pause for a moment at the top.
- **Lower Arms:** Gradually lower your arms back to the starting position in a controlled manner.

- **Repeat:** Perform 10-15 repetitions, maintaining good form throughout the exercise.

Tips for Overhead Arm Lifts:

- Engage your core to support your lower back.
- Move slowly and avoid using momentum to lift the weights.
- If using weights is too challenging, start with just the arm movements and gradually add resistance as you become stronger.

c. Bicep Curls with a Resistance Band

Bicep curls with a resistance band are an excellent way to strengthen the biceps and improve overall arm strength. Resistance bands offer adjustable resistance, making them ideal for various fitness levels.

How to Do Bicep Curls with a Resistance Band:

1. **Starting Position:** Sit up straight with your feet flat on the floor, about shoulder-width apart. Place the center of the resistance band under your feet, holding one end of the band in each hand with your arms hanging down by your sides.
2. **Grip:** Ensure that your palms are facing forward, and your elbows are close to your body.
3. **Curl:** Slowly bend your elbows and curl your hands towards your shoulders, keeping your upper arms stationary. Focus on contracting your biceps as you lift.
4. **Pause and Squeeze:** Hold the position for a second, squeezing your biceps at the top of the movement.
5. **Lower:** Gradually lower your hands back to the starting position in a controlled manner.
6. **Repeat:** Perform 10-15 repetitions, focusing on the contraction of the biceps during each curl.

Tips for Bicep Curls with a Resistance Band:

- Keep your wrists straight and avoid bending them during the curl.
- Maintain a steady and controlled pace, avoiding jerky movements.

- Adjust the resistance by changing the length of the band under your feet or by using bands with different resistance levels.

d. Triceps Dips Using a Chair

Triceps dips are a powerful exercise for strengthening the triceps, shoulders, and chest. Using a chair for this exercise makes it accessible and effective for building upper body strength.

How to Do Triceps Dips Using a Chair:

- **Starting Position:** Sit on the edge of a sturdy chair with your hands gripping the front edge of the seat, fingers pointing forward. Your feet should be flat on the floor, about hip-width apart.
- **Move Off the Chair:** Slide your buttocks off the chair, supporting your weight with your hands. Your knees should be bent at a 90-degree angle, and your feet should be securely planted on the ground.
- **Lower Your Body:** Slowly bend your elbows to lower your body to the floor. Keep your back against the chair and your elbows pointed straight back. Lower your elbows until they create a 90-degree angle.
- **Lift Your Body:** Press through your palms to straighten your arms and lift your body back to the starting position.
- **Repeat:** Perform 8-12 repetitions, focusing on the contraction of the triceps during each dip.

Tips for Triceps Dips Using a Chair

Triceps dips using a chair are a great exercise for targeting the triceps and improving upper body strength. Here's how to perform them correctly and safely:

1. Choose the Right Chair

- **Sturdy Chair:** Ensure the chair is stable and can support your weight. A heavy-duty, solid chair with no wheels is ideal.

- **Flat Surface:** Place the chair on a flat, non-slippery surface to prevent it from moving during the exercise.

2. Proper Positioning

- **Seat Depth:** Sit on the edge of the chair with your hands next to your hips, fingers facing forward or slightly inward. Your feet should be level on the floor, with your knees bent 90 degrees.
- **Hand Placement:** Place your hands on the edge of the seat, ensuring your fingers are pointing forward and your palms are flat. Your hands should be around shoulder width apart.

3. Performing the Dip

- **Starting Position:** Move your hips forward off the chair, keeping your buttocks close to the seat. Support your body weight with your arms.
- **Lowering:** Bend your elbows slowly and lower your body down toward the floor. Keep your elbows tight to your body and don't allow them to flare out to the side.
- **Depth:** Lower yourself until your upper arms are parallel to the floor or slightly below, depending on your comfort and flexibility.
- **Pushing Up:** Push through your palms and straighten your elbows to lift your body back to the starting position. Engage your triceps throughout the movement.

4. Form and Technique

- **Keep Core Engaged:** Maintain a tight core throughout the exercise to stabilize your body and protect your lower back.
- **Avoid Shoulder Shrugging:** Keep your shoulders down and away from your ears to avoid unnecessary strain on the shoulder joints.
- **Control the Movement:** Perform the exercise with a controlled tempo to maximize muscle engagement and minimize the risk of injury.

5. Safety Considerations

- **Warm Up:** Perform a thorough warm-up before doing triceps dips to prepare your muscles and joints.
- **Check for Discomfort:** If you experience sharp pain or discomfort in your shoulders or wrists, stop and reassess your form or consider alternative exercises.
- **Modify if Needed:** If you're a beginner or have limited strength, you can start by bending your knees and keeping your feet closer to the chair to reduce the amount of body weight you're lifting.

6. Variations for Progression

- **Straight Leg Variation:** For more challenge, extend your legs straight out in front of you while performing the dip.
- **Weighted Dips:** Once you're comfortable with bodyweight dips, you can add resistance by placing a weight on your lap or using a weighted vest.

By following these tips, you can effectively perform triceps dips using a chair while minimizing the risk of injury and maximizing the exercise's benefits.

Chapter 3: Lower Body Workouts

Maintaining lower body strength is essential for overall mobility, balance, and independence, particularly as we age. This chapter focuses on exercises that target the legs and lower body, which can be performed while seated or with the support of a chair. The exercises covered in this chapter are Seated Leg Lifts, Chair Squats, Knee Raises, Calf Raises, and

Ankle Rotations. Each exercise is designed to enhance strength, flexibility, and circulation in the lower body.

a. Seated Leg Lifts

Seated leg lifts are excellent for strengthening the quadriceps, hip flexors, and core muscles. This exercise improves leg strength and mobility, making daily activities easier.

How to Do Seated Leg Lifts:

- **Starting Position:** Sit up straight in a sturdy chair with your feet flat on the floor and your hands resting on the sides of the chair for support.
- **Lift One Leg:** Slowly lift your right leg straight out in front of you, keeping your knee slightly bent. Lift the leg as high as you comfortably can without leaning back.
- **Hold:** Hold the lifted position for a few seconds, feeling the contraction in your thigh muscles.
- **Lower:** Gradually lower your leg back to the starting position.
- **Repeat:** Perform 10-15 repetitions with the right leg, then switch to the left leg and repeat.

Tips for Seated Leg Lifts:

- Keep your back straight and avoid leaning back during the lift.
- Move slowly and with control to maximize muscle engagement.
- If the exercise is too challenging, start with shorter lifts and gradually increase the height as you gain strength.

b. Chair Squats

Chair squats are a modified version of traditional squats, providing a great way to strengthen the quadriceps, hamstrings, glutes, and core. This exercise also helps improve balance and functional mobility.

How to Do Chair Squats:

- **Starting Position:** Stand in front of a sturdy chair with your feet shoulder-width apart and your toes pointing slightly outward.
- **Lower into the Chair:** Slowly lower your body towards the chair as if you are about to sit down. Keep your chest up and your back straight. Your knees should bend and move slightly forward, but not past your toes.
- **Touch the Chair:** Lightly touch the chair with your buttocks, but do not sit down completely.
- **Stand Up:** Press through your heels to stand back up to the starting position, straightening your legs fully.
- **Repeat:** Perform 10-15 repetitions, maintaining good form throughout the exercise.

Tips for Chair Squats:

- Keep your weight on your heels and avoid shifting forward onto your toes.
- Engage your core muscles to support your lower back.
- Use the chair as a guide to maintain proper depth and form.

c. Knee Raises

Knee raises are an effective exercise for strengthening the hip flexors, lower abdominal muscles, and quadriceps. This exercise also helps improve coordination and balance.

How to Do Knee Raises:

- **Starting Position:** Sit up straight in a sturdy chair with your feet flat on the floor and your hands resting on the sides of the chair for support.
- **Lift One Knee:** Slowly lift your right knee towards your chest, keeping your back straight and your abdominal muscles engaged.
- **Hold:** Hold the lifted position for a few seconds, feeling the contraction in your hip flexors and lower abs.
- **Lower:** Gradually lower your knee back to the starting position.
- **Repeat:** Perform 10-15 repetitions with the right knee, then switch to the left knee and repeat.

Tips for Knee Raises:

- Maintain a neutral spine and avoid leaning back during the lift.
- To get the most out of your muscles, use controlled motions.
- If the exercise is too challenging, start with smaller lifts and gradually increase the height as you gain strength.

d. Calf Raises

Calf raises are a basic yet efficient calf muscle building exercise. Strong calves improve balance, support the ankle joints, and enhance overall lower body stability.

How to Do Calf Raises:

- **Starting Position:** Sit up straight in a sturdy chair with your feet flat on the floor and your hands resting on the sides of the chair for support.
- **Lift Heels:** Slowly lift your heels off the floor, rising onto the balls of your feet. Focus on contracting your calf muscles as you lift.
- **Hold:** Hold the lifted position for a few seconds, feeling the contraction in your calves.
- **Lower:** Gradually lower your heels back to the starting position.
- **Repeat:** Perform 10-15 repetitions, maintaining good form throughout the exercise.

Tips for Calf Raises:

- Keep your movements controlled and avoid bouncing.
- Engage your core to support your lower back.
- If the exercise is too easy, try performing it while standing and holding onto the back of the chair for balance.

e. Ankle Rotations

Ankle rotations are a great exercise for improving flexibility and circulation in the lower legs and ankles. This exercise helps maintain ankle mobility and can reduce the risk of sprains and stiffness.

How to Do Ankle Rotations:

- **Starting Position:** Sit up straight in a sturdy chair with your feet flat on the floor and your hands resting on the sides of the chair for support.
- **Lift One Foot:** Lift your right foot off the floor and extend your leg slightly.
- **Rotate Ankle:** Slowly rotate your ankle in a circular motion, making full circles. Perform the rotations in one direction for about 10-15 seconds, then reverse the direction.
- **Lower Foot:** Gradually lower your foot back to the starting position.
- **Repeat:** Perform 10-15 rotations in each direction with the right ankle, then switch to the left ankle and repeat.

Tips for Ankle Rotations:

- Keep the movements slow and controlled to maximize flexibility and circulation.
- Avoid making jerky or fast movements to prevent strain.
- If you experience discomfort, reduce the range of motion or take a break.

Conclusion

Lower body strength is vital for overall health, mobility, and independence. Seated Leg Lifts, Chair Squats, Knee Raises, Calf Raises, and Ankle Rotations are effective exercises that target the legs and lower body. These exercises can be performed safely while seated or with the support of a chair, making them accessible for mature individuals and those with mobility challenges. By incorporating these exercises into your routine, you can enhance your strength, flexibility, and circulation, supporting an active and independent lifestyle.

Chapter 4: Core Strengthening

A strong core is essential for balance, stability, and overall functional fitness. The core muscles, which include the abdominals, obliques, and lower back muscles, play a vital role in almost every movement we make. This chapter focuses on core strengthening exercises that can be performed while seated. The exercises covered are Seated Torso Twists, Seated Crunches, Oblique Twists, Seated Side Bends, and Pelvic Tilts. These exercises help improve core strength, stability, and posture, contributing to better overall health and mobility.

a. Seated Torso Twists

Seated torso twists are excellent for engaging the oblique muscles and improving spinal flexibility. This exercise helps enhance rotational strength, which is crucial for daily activities that involve twisting movements.

How to Do Seated Torso Twists:

- **Starting Position:** Sit up straight in a sturdy chair with your feet flat on the floor and your hands resting on your thighs.
- **Twist to One Side:** Place your right hand on the back of the chair and your left hand on your right thigh. Gently twist your torso to the right, leading with your shoulders and looking over your right shoulder.

- **Hold:** Hold the twist for a few seconds, feeling the stretch in your obliques and spine.
- **Return to Center:** Slowly return to the starting position.
- **Repeat on the Other Side:** Perform the twist to the left side, placing your left hand on the back of the chair and your right hand on your left thigh. Hold the twist for a few seconds and return to the center.
- **Repeat:** Perform 10-15 repetitions on each side, focusing on controlled movements.

Tips for Seated Torso Twists:

- Keep your back straight and avoid slouching during the twist.
- Move slowly and avoid jerky movements to prevent strain.
- Breathe deeply and steadily throughout the exercise.

b. Seated Crunches

Seated crunches target the upper abdominals and help strengthen the core muscles. This exercise mimics the traditional crunch but is performed in a seated position, making it accessible for those with mobility issues.

How to Do Seated Crunches:

7. **Starting Position:** Sit up straight in a sturdy chair with your feet flat on the floor and your hands resting behind your head, elbows pointing out to the sides.
8. **Engage Core:** Engage your abdominal muscles by pulling your belly button towards your spine.
9. **Crunch Forward:** Slowly curl your upper body forward, bringing your chest towards your thighs. Focus on contracting your abdominals as you curl.
10. **Hold:** Hold the crunch position for a second, squeezing your abdominals.
11. **Return to Starting Position:** Gradually return to the starting position, keeping your core engaged.
12. **Repeat:** Perform 10-15 repetitions, maintaining good form throughout the exercise.

Tips for Seated Crunches:

- Avoid pulling on your neck with your hands; use your core muscles to lift your torso.
- To get the most out of the workout, move gently and deliberately.
- Breathe out as you crunch forward and inhale as you return to the starting position.

c. Oblique Twists

Oblique twists specifically target the oblique muscles, which are essential for rotational movements and maintaining a strong core. This exercise helps enhance flexibility and strength in the sides of the torso.

How to Do Oblique Twists:

- **Starting Position:** Sit up straight in a sturdy chair with your feet flat on the floor and your hands holding a light weight or a water bottle in front of your chest.
- **Twist to One Side:** Engage your core and slowly twist your torso to the right, keeping your arms at chest level and moving together with your torso.
- **Return to Center:** Return to the starting position, maintaining control.
- **Twist to the Other Side:** Perform the twist to the left side, ensuring your movements are slow and controlled.
- **Repeat:** Perform 10-15 repetitions on each side, focusing on engaging the oblique muscles.

Tips for Oblique Twists:

- Keep your back straight and avoid slouching during the twist.
- Use your core muscles to control the movement, not just your arms.

- Begin with a small weight, gradually increasing the resistance as you gain strength.

d. Seated Side Bends

Seated side bends target the obliques and help improve lateral flexibility and strength. This exercise is beneficial for enhancing core stability and reducing the risk of injury.

How to Do Seated Side Bends:

- **Starting Position:** Sit up straight in a sturdy chair with your feet flat on the floor and your hands resting on your thighs.
- **Bend to One Side:** Raise your right arm overhead and slowly bend your torso to the left, reaching towards the floor with your left hand. Keep your right arm in line with your ear.
- **Hold:** Hold the side bend for a few seconds, feeling the stretch in your right side.
- **Return to Center:** Gradually return to the starting position.
- **Repeat on the Other Side:** Raise your left arm overhead and perform the side bend to the right, holding for a few seconds before returning to the center.
- **Repeat:** Perform 10-15 repetitions on each side, focusing on controlled movements.

Tips for Seated Side Bends:

- Keep your back straight and avoid slouching during the bend.
- Move slowly and avoid jerky movements to prevent strain.
- Breathe deeply and steadily throughout the exercise.

e. Pelvic Tilts

Pelvic tilts are an excellent exercise for strengthening the lower abdominals and lower back muscles. This exercise helps improve core stability and can alleviate lower back pain.

How to Do Pelvic Tilts:

- **Starting Position:** Sit up straight in a sturdy chair with your feet flat on the floor and your hands resting on your thighs.
- **Tilt Pelvis Forward:** Slowly tilt your pelvis forward, arching your lower back slightly. Focus on engaging your lower abdominal muscles.
- **Hold:** Hold the tilt for a few seconds, feeling the contraction in your lower abdominals.
- **Tilt Pelvis Back:** Gradually tilt your pelvis back, flattening your lower back against the chair. Focus on squeezing your glutes and lower abdominals.
- **Hold:** Hold the tilt for a few seconds before returning to the starting position.
- **Repeat:** Perform 10-15 repetitions, maintaining good form throughout the exercise.

Tips for Pelvic Tilts:

- Keep your upper body still and focus on the movement in your pelvis.
- To get the most out of the workout, move gently and deliberately.
- Breathe deeply and steadily throughout the exercise.

Conclusion

Strengthening the core is crucial for overall health, stability, and mobility. Seated Torso Twists, Seated Crunches, Oblique Twists, Seated Side Bends, and Pelvic Tilts are effective exercises that target the core muscles and can be performed safely while seated. These exercises help improve core strength, stability, and posture, contributing to better overall health and functional fitness. By incorporating these exercises into your routine, you can enhance your core strength and enjoy the benefits of a strong, stable, and flexible core.

Chapter 5: Flexibility and Stretching

Maintaining flexibility is essential for overall mobility, reducing the risk of injury, and promoting relaxation. This chapter focuses on flexibility and stretching exercises that can be performed while seated. The exercises covered are Deep Breathing Techniques, Neck Stretches, Shoulder

Stretches, Seated Hamstring Stretch, Ankle Flex and Stretch, and Wrist and Forearm Stretches. These exercises help improve flexibility, reduce tension, and enhance overall well-being.

a. Deep Breathing Techniques

Deep breathing techniques are fundamental for relaxation and can enhance the effectiveness of stretching exercises. Proper breathing helps oxygenate the muscles and promotes a sense of calm.

How to Practice Deep Breathing:

- **Starting Position:** Sit up straight in a sturdy chair with your feet flat on the floor and your hands resting on your thighs.
- **Inhale Deeply:** Take a steady, deep breath in through your nose, allowing your belly to expand as you fill your lungs with oxygen.
- **Hold:** Hold your breath for a few seconds.
- **Exhale Slowly:** Exhale slowly through your mouth, letting your abdomen contract as you release the air.
- **Repeat:** Perform this deep breathing exercise for 5-10 breaths, focusing on relaxation and proper technique.

b. Neck Stretches

Neck stretches help alleviate tension and improve flexibility in the neck and upper shoulders. This exercise is beneficial for reducing stiffness and promoting better posture.

How to Do Neck Stretches:

- **Starting Position:** Sit up straight with your feet flat on the floor and your hands resting on your thighs.
- **Tilt to One Side:** Gently tilt your head to the right, bringing your right ear towards your right shoulder. Hold the stretch for 15-20 seconds.
- **Return to Center:** Slowly return to the starting position.
- **Tilt to the Other Side:** Repeat the stretch on the left side, holding for 15-20 seconds.

- **Repeat:** Perform 2-3 repetitions on each side.

c. Shoulder Stretches

Shoulder stretches are effective for improving flexibility and reducing tension in the shoulders and upper back. This exercise helps enhance range of motion and relieve stress.

How to Do Shoulder Stretches:

- **Starting Position:** Sit up straight with your feet flat on the floor and your hands resting on your thighs.
- **Cross Arm Stretch:** Bring your right arm across your chest and use your left hand to gently pull your right arm closer to your body. Hold the stretch for 15-20 seconds.
- **Switch Sides:** Repeat the stretch with your left arm, holding for 15-20 seconds.
- **Repeat:** Perform 2-3 repetitions on each side.

d. Seated Hamstring Stretch

The seated hamstring stretches targets the muscles in the back of the thigh. This exercise helps improve flexibility in the hamstrings and lower back.

How to Do Seated Hamstring Stretch:

- **Starting Position:** Sit on the edge of a sturdy chair with your feet flat on the floor and your hands resting on your thighs.
- **Extend One Leg:** Extend your right leg straight out in front of you, resting your heel on the floor.
- **Lean Forward:** Gently lean forward from your hips, reaching towards your right foot. Maintain a straight back and prevent curving the spine.
- **Hold:** Hold the stretch for 15-20 seconds, feeling the stretch in your hamstring.
- **Switch Sides:** Repeat the stretch with your left leg, holding for 15-20 seconds.
- **Repeat:** Perform 2-3 repetitions on each side.

e. Ankle Flex and Stretch

Ankle flex and stretch exercises improve flexibility and circulation in the ankles and lower legs. This exercise helps maintain ankle mobility and reduce the risk of stiffness.

How to Do Ankle Flex and Stretch:

- **Starting Position:** Sit up straight with your feet flat on the floor and your hands resting on your thighs.
- **Lift One Foot:** Lift your right foot off the floor and extend your leg slightly.
- **Flex and Point:** Flex your foot by pulling your toes towards your shin, then point your toes away from your body. Perform this movement slowly and with control.
- **Repeat:** Perform 10-15 repetitions with your right ankle, then switch to your left ankle and repeat.

f. Wrist and Forearm Stretches

Wrist and forearm stretch help reduce tension and improve flexibility in the wrists and forearms. This exercise is particularly beneficial for those who spend a lot of time typing or using their hands.

How to Do Wrist and Forearm Stretches:

13. **Starting Position:** Sit up straight with your feet flat on the floor and your hands resting on your thighs.
14. **Extend One Arm:** Extend your right arm in front of you with your palm facing up.
15. **Stretch Fingers:** Use your left hand to gently pull back on your right fingers, stretching the wrist and forearm. Hold the stretch for 15-20 seconds.
16. **Switch Sides:** Repeat the stretch with your left arm, holding for 15-20 seconds.
17. **Repeat:** Perform 2-3 repetitions on each side.

Conclusion

Flexibility and stretching are crucial components of a balanced fitness routine, especially for maintaining mobility and reducing the risk of injury. Deep Breathing Techniques, Neck Stretches, Shoulder Stretches, Seated Hamstring Stretch, Ankle Flex and Stretch, and Wrist and Forearm Stretches are effective exercises that can be performed while seated. These exercises help improve flexibility, reduce tension, and enhance overall well-being, contributing to a healthier and more active lifestyle. By incorporating these stretches into your routine, you can enjoy greater flexibility, relaxation, and improved physical function.

Chapter 6: Cardiovascular Seated Workouts

Maintaining cardiovascular health is essential for overall well-being, energy levels, and longevity. Even while seated, you can perform exercises that get your heart rate up and improve cardiovascular fitness. This chapter focuses on seated cardiovascular workouts, which are designed to elevate your heart rate and enhance endurance. The exercises covered are Seated Jumping Jacks, Seated Jogging, Arm Punches, Seated Tap Dance, and Speedy Leg Lifts. These exercises are ideal for individuals with limited mobility or those who prefer low-impact workouts.

a. Seated Jumping Jacks

Seated jumping jacks mimic the movement of traditional jumping jacks but are performed while seated. This exercise helps improve cardiovascular health and coordination.

How to Do Seated Jumping Jacks:

- **Starting Position:** Sit up straight in a sturdy chair with your feet flat on the floor and your arms at your sides.
- **Extend Arms and Legs:** Simultaneously extend your arms out to the sides and your legs out to the sides, mimicking the jumping jack movement.
- **Return to Center:** Bring your arms back to your sides and your feet back together.
- **Repeat:** Perform this movement continuously for 1-2 minutes, keeping a steady pace.
- **Tips for Seated Jumping Jacks:**
- Maintain a straight back and avoid slouching.
- Move your arms and legs simultaneously for a coordinated movement.
- Keep breathing steadily throughout the exercise.

b. Seated Jogging

Seated jogging is a low-impact way to simulate jogging while remaining seated. This exercise increases heart rate and improves cardiovascular endurance.

How to Do Seated Jogging:

- **Starting Position:** Sit up straight in a sturdy chair with your feet flat on the floor and your arms bent at a 90-degree angle at your sides.
- **Jog in Place:** Alternate lifting your feet off the floor as if you are jogging, while simultaneously moving your arms back and forth.
- **Maintain Pace:** Keep a steady pace, moving your arms and legs rhythmically.

- **Duration:** Perform this movement for 1-2 minutes, aiming to keep a consistent pace.

Tips for Seated Jogging:

- Engage your core to maintain good posture.
- Focus on lifting your knees and swinging your arms in sync.
- Breathe steadily and rhythmically.

c. Arm Punches

Arm punches are a great way to get your heart rate up while also working your upper body. This exercise targets the shoulders, arms, and chest muscles.

How to Do Arm Punches:

- **Starting Position:** Sit up straight in a sturdy chair with your feet flat on the floor and your hands in fists at chest level.
- **Punch Forward:** Extend your right arm forward in a punching motion, then bring it back to your chest.
- **Alternate Arms:** Repeat the punching motion with your left arm.
- **Continuous Movement:** Alternate punches continuously for 1-2 minutes, maintaining a steady rhythm.

Tips for Arm Punches:

- Keep your movements controlled and avoid locking your elbows.
- Engage your core and maintain a straight back.
- Focus on breathing steadily and maintaining a rhythm.

d. Seated Tap Dance

Seated tap dance involves rhythmic foot movements that mimic tap dancing. This exercise is fun and effective for improving cardiovascular fitness and coordination.

How to Do Seated Tap Dance:

- **Starting Position:** Sit up straight in a sturdy chair with your feet flat on the floor.
- **Tap Feet:** Alternate tapping your toes and heels on the floor, mimicking a tap dance movement.
- **Add Arm Movements:** For added intensity, move your arms in a rhythmic pattern, such as swinging them side to side.
- **Duration:** Perform this movement for 1-2 minutes, keeping a steady rhythm.

Tips for Seated Tap Dance:

- Maintain good posture and engage your core.
- Keep your movements rhythmic and controlled.
- Enjoy the music and let it guide your pace.

e. Speedy Leg Lifts

Speedy leg lifts are a more vigorous version of seated leg lifts, focusing on rapid movement to elevate the heart rate. This exercise targets the lower body and core muscles.

How to Do Speedy Leg Lifts:

- **Starting Position:** Sit up straight in a sturdy chair with your feet flat on the floor and your hands resting on the sides of the chair for support.
- **Lift Legs Rapidly:** Quickly lift your right leg straight out in front of you, then lower it and immediately lift your left leg.
- **Alternate Legs:** Continue alternating leg lifts rapidly, maintaining a fast pace.
- **Duration:** Perform this movement for 1-2 minutes, aiming to keep a consistent pace.

Tips for Speedy Leg Lifts:

- Keep your back straight and avoid leaning back.
- Move your legs rapidly but with control to avoid strain.
- Breathe steadily and focus on maintaining a fast rhythm.

Conclusion

Cardiovascular health is crucial for maintaining overall fitness and energy levels. Seated Jumping Jacks, Seated Jogging, Arm Punches, Seated Tap Dance, and Speedy Leg Lifts are effective exercises that can be performed while seated, making them accessible for individuals with limited mobility. These exercises help elevate the heart rate, improve endurance, and enhance cardiovascular fitness. By incorporating these workouts into your routine, you can enjoy the benefits of a healthy heart and an active lifestyle, even while sitting down.

Chapter 7: Combining Workouts into Routines

Creating structured workout routines can help you stay consistent and ensure that you're targeting different muscle groups effectively. This chapter provides a guide for combining the exercises discussed into cohesive 10-minute routines. These routines are designed to be quick, effective, and adaptable to your fitness level and goals. The routines covered are the 10-Minute Upper Body Routine, 10-Minute Lower Body Routine, 10-Minute Full Body Routine, 10-Minute Cardio Routine, and 10-Minute Flexibility Routine.

a. 10-Minute Upper Body Routine

This routine focuses on strengthening and toning the muscles of the upper body, including the arms, shoulders, and chest.

Routine Breakdown:

- **Warm-Up (1 minute):** Arm circles and shoulder shrugs to get the blood flowing.
- **Overhead Arm Lifts (2 minutes):** Perform slow and controlled overhead arm lifts, engaging your shoulder muscles.
- **Bicep Curls with Resistance Band (2 minutes):** Use a resistance band to perform bicep curls, focusing on controlled movements.
- **Triceps Dips Using a Chair (2 minutes):** Use the edge of your chair to perform triceps dips, targeting the back of your arms.
- **Arm Punches (2 minutes):** Alternate rapid arm punches to get your heart rate up and work your shoulders and chest.
- **Cool Down (1 minute):** Shoulder stretches to relax the muscles and improve flexibility.

Tips:

- Use light weights or resistance bands for added intensity.
- Focus on controlled movements to prevent injury.

b. 10-Minute Lower Body Routine

This routine targets the muscles of the lower body, including the thighs, hamstrings, and calves.

Routine Breakdown:

- **Warm-Up (1 minute):** Gentle seated marching to warm up the legs.

- **Seated Leg Lifts (2 minutes):** Perform alternating leg lifts, focusing on engaging your thigh muscles.
- **Chair Squats (2 minutes):** Stand up from and sit back down on the chair repeatedly, ensuring controlled movements.
- **Knee Raises (2 minutes):** Lift your knees towards your chest alternately, engaging your core and hip flexors.
- **Calf Raises (2 minutes):** Lift your heels off the ground and lower them back down to work your calf muscles.
- **Cool Down (1 minute):** Ankle rotations to relax and stretch the lower leg muscles.

Tips:

- Ensure your chair is stable and secure.
- Move at your own pace to maintain balance and control.

c. 10-Minute Full Body Routine

This routine is designed to give a balanced workout, engaging both upper and lower body muscles along with some core exercises.

Routine Breakdown:

- **Warm-Up (1 minute):** Gentle seated marching.
- **Overhead Arm Lifts (1.5 minutes):** Engage your shoulder muscles with controlled overhead lifts.
- **Seated Leg Lifts (1.5 minutes):** Strengthen your lower body with alternating leg lifts.
- **Seated Torso Twists (1.5 minutes):** Improve core strength and flexibility with torso twists.
- **Arm Punches (1.5 minutes):** Get your heart rate up and work your upper body.
- **Chair Squats (1.5 minutes):** Strengthen your legs and glutes with controlled chair squats.
- **Cool Down (1 minute):** Deep breathing and shoulder stretches.
- **Tips:**
- Focus on smooth, controlled movements.
- Modify exercises as needed to suit your fitness level.

d. 10-Minute Cardio Routine

This routine is designed to get your heart rate up and improve cardiovascular fitness.

Routine Breakdown:

- **Warm-Up (1 minute):** Gentle seated marching.
- **Seated Jumping Jacks (2 minutes):** Mimic the motion of jumping jacks to elevate your heart rate.
- **Seated Jogging (2 minutes):** Alternate lifting your feet off the floor as if jogging, while moving your arms.
- **Seated Tap Dance (2 minutes):** Tap your toes and heels rhythmically, adding arm movements for intensity.
- **Speedy Leg Lifts (2 minutes):** Rapidly alternate leg lifts to keep your heart rate up.
- **Cool Down (1 minute):** Deep breathing and gentle stretching.

Tips:

- Maintain a steady pace and breathe regularly.
- Use music to help keep rhythm and motivation.

e. 10-Minute Flexibility Routine

This routine focuses on stretching and improving flexibility in various muscle groups.

Routine Breakdown:

- **Warm-Up (1 minute):** Deep breathing techniques to relax and prepare for stretching.
- **Neck Stretches (2 minutes):** Gently stretch the muscles in your neck and shoulders.
- **Shoulder Stretches (2 minutes):** Perform cross-arm stretches to improve shoulder flexibility.
- **Seated Hamstring Stretch (2 minutes):** Stretch the back of your thighs with controlled hamstring stretches.

- **Ankle Flex and Stretch (2 minutes):** Improve ankle flexibility with flexing and pointing movements.
- **Wrist and Forearm Stretches (1 minute):** Stretch your wrists and forearms to reduce tension and improve flexibility.

Tips:

- Hold each stretch for at least 15-20 seconds.
- Breathe deeply and relax into each stretch.

Conclusion

Combining the various exercises into structured routines helps ensure you get a balanced and effective workout. These 10-minute routines are designed to be quick and easy to fit into your daily schedule, promoting consistency and long-term fitness benefits. By integrating these routines into your regular exercise regimen, you can enjoy improved strength, flexibility, and cardiovascular health while remaining seated.

Chapter 8: Special Considerations

Incorporating exercise into daily routines is crucial for overall health, but special considerations must be considered for individuals with specific conditions. This chapter focuses on tailoring exercise regimens for those with arthritis, osteoporosis, heart health concerns, and emphasizes low-impact variations to ensure safety and effectiveness.

a. Exercises for Arthritis

Arthritis, characterized by joint inflammation, pain, and stiffness, requires a careful approach to exercise to prevent exacerbation of symptoms. Low-impact activities are often recommended to minimize joint stress.

- **Range-of-Motion Exercises:** These exercises help you stay flexible and minimize stiffness. Gentle stretching and movements such as arm circles, knee bends, and ankle rotations are beneficial. Incorporating activities like tai chi or gentle yoga can also improve joint function and reduce pain.
- **Strength Training:** Using light weights or resistance bands can help strengthen the muscles around affected joints, providing better support and stability. Exercises like seated leg lifts, wall push-ups, and bicep curls can be effective while minimizing joint strain.
- **Aerobic Exercise:** Low-impact aerobic exercises, such as swimming, water aerobics, and cycling, are excellent choices. They improve cardiovascular health and overall fitness without putting undue pressure on the joints.
- **Flexibility and Balance Training:** Incorporating exercises that enhance flexibility and balance, such as stretching routines and balance exercises like standing on one foot, can improve mobility and prevent falls.

b. Exercises for Osteoporosis

Osteoporosis, characterized by weakened bones and an increased risk of fractures, requires a focus on bone-strengthening activities. Maintaining bone density requires weight-bearing and resistance activities.

- **Weight-Bearing Exercises:** Activities like walking, dancing, and hiking are beneficial as they force the bones to support the body's weight, stimulating bone growth.
- **Resistance Training:** Using weights or resistance bands can enhance bone density by stressing the bones through muscle contractions. Exercises such as squats, lunges, and resistance band rows are recommended.
- **Balance and Stability Exercises:** To prevent falls, which can lead to fractures, balance exercises are crucial. Practices like standing on one leg, heel-to-toe walking, and balance exercises on unstable surfaces can improve stability.
- **Low-Impact Options:** For individuals with advanced osteoporosis, focusing on low-impact activities like water aerobics and chair exercises can provide cardiovascular benefits while minimizing fracture risk.

c. Exercises for Heart Health

Maintaining cardiovascular health involves exercises that improve heart function and overall fitness. It's essential to focus on both aerobic and strength training exercises, considering any specific cardiovascular conditions.

- **Aerobic Exercise:** Regular aerobic activities, such as brisk walking, jogging, cycling, and swimming, help strengthen the heart muscle, improve circulation, and reduce blood pressure. The goal is to engage in at least 150 minutes (about 2 and a half hours) of moderate-intensity aerobic exercise per week.
- **Strength Training:** Incorporating moderate strength training exercises, such as body-weight exercises (e.g., squats, push-ups) and resistance bands, can improve muscular strength and support heart health. Aim for at least two days a week of strength training.

- **Flexibility and Stretching:** Regular stretching exercises can improve overall flexibility, reducing the risk of injuries and aiding in recovery Practices such as yoga and Pilates might be very effective.
- **Interval Training:** For those who are already active, incorporating high-intensity interval training (HIIT) can further enhance cardiovascular fitness. This entails alternating short bursts of high-intensity activity with intervals of low-intensity exercise.

d. Low-Impact Variations

Low-impact exercises are beneficial for individuals who need to minimize joint stress or manage chronic conditions. They can be adapted for various fitness levels and health conditions.

- **Water-Based Exercises:** Swimming and water aerobics provide a full-body workout while reducing joint impact, making them ideal for individuals with arthritis or joint pain.
- **Stationary Cycling:** Cycling on a stationary bike offers a cardiovascular workout that is easy on the knees and hips. It also helps build leg strength and endurance.
- **Chair Exercises:** For those with mobility issues, chair exercises can be a safe and effective way to stay active. These exercises can include seated leg lifts, seated marches, and seated arm exercises.
- **Gentle Yoga and Pilates:** Both yoga and Pilates offer low-impact options that improve flexibility, strength, and balance without putting excessive stress on the joints.

By tailoring exercise routines to accommodate specific health conditions and focusing on low-impact options, individuals can safely and effectively enhance their overall well-being and maintain a healthy lifestyle.

Chapter 9: Adapting Workouts for Different Abilities

Adapting workouts to accommodate different abilities ensures inclusivity and effectiveness. This chapter focuses on modifying exercises for individuals with limited mobility and offers practical adaptations to make exercise accessible for everyone.

a. Modifying Exercises for Limited Mobility

When addressing limited mobility, it's essential to provide modifications that enhance accessibility without compromising the effectiveness of the workout.

a. Using Resistance Bands and Weights

- **Resistance Bands:** Resistance bands are versatile tools that can be used to perform a wide range of exercises. They provide adjustable resistance and can be utilized in various positions, including seated or lying down. For individuals with limited mobility, bands can be anchored to a chair or a sturdy surface to perform exercises such as seated bicep curls, chest presses, and leg lifts. Their flexibility allows for controlled movements and reduces the risk of injury.
- **Weights:** Light weights or dumbbells can be used to perform strength training exercises with adaptations for limited mobility. For example, seated exercises such as shoulder presses, lateral raises, and seated rows can be done while sitting in a chair. Using weights in this manner helps build strength and maintain muscle mass. Individuals can also use weight vests or ankle weights for additional resistance while performing exercises like seated marches or leg lifts.

b. Chair Yoga Adaptations

Chair yoga offers a range of adaptations that make yoga accessible to those with limited mobility. It allows individuals to perform yoga postures and stretches while seated, providing support and stability.

- **Seated Poses:** Many traditional yoga poses can be adapted for a seated position. For example, seated forward bends, gentle twists, and seated side stretches can be performed while sitting in a sturdy chair. These adaptations help improve flexibility, balance, and relaxation without requiring the individual to move to the floor.
- **Standing Poses with Chair Support:** For those who can stand but need support, using a chair for balance can allow for modified standing poses. Poses like chair-supported warrior or tree pose can be adapted by holding onto the back of a chair for stability, thus providing a safer way to build strength and balance.
- **Breathing and Relaxation:** Chair yoga is also beneficial for incorporating breathing exercises and relaxation techniques. Practices such as diaphragmatic breathing, seated meditation, and

gentle stretching can be done while seated to promote relaxation and mental well-being.

Chapter 10: Staying Motivated

Maintaining motivation is critical to long-term success in any fitness program. This chapter provides strategies to set realistic goals, track progress, overcome plateaus, and stay consistent.

a. Setting Realistic Goals

Setting achievable and realistic goals is foundational to maintaining motivation. Goals should be specific, measurable, attainable, relevant, and time-bound (SMART). Start with short-term goals, such as completing a certain number of workouts per week, and progress to long-term goals, like achieving a specific fitness milestone. By setting clear, manageable goals, individuals can maintain focus and celebrate their progress along the way.

b. Tracking Progress

Tracking progress helps in assessing improvements and staying motivated. Use fitness journals, apps, or spreadsheets to record workouts, track achievements, and note any changes in physical abilities or health metrics. Regularly reviewing this progress can provide a sense of accomplishment and highlight areas for further improvement. Additionally, tracking progress helps in adjusting goals and workouts as needed.

c. Overcoming Plateaus

Plateaus are a common challenge in fitness journeys. To overcome them, vary workouts to introduce new challenges and prevent boredom. This might involve changing exercise routines, increasing intensity, or incorporating different types of physical activities. Additionally, evaluating diet, rest, and recovery can help identify factors contributing to the plateau and provide opportunities for adjustment.

d. Staying Consistent

Consistency is key to achieving long-term fitness goals. Establish a regular workout schedule and incorporate exercise into daily routines. Find activities that are enjoyable and align with personal preferences to make adherence easier. Engaging with a workout buddy or joining a fitness community can provide additional support and accountability, further enhancing motivation and consistency.

Chapter 11: Resources and References

Providing additional resources and references helps readers access further information and support for their fitness journey.

a. Recommended Equipment and Gear

- **Resistance Bands:** Adjustable and portable, these bands are ideal for strength training and flexibility exercises. They have different resistance levels and may be used for a variety of activities.
- **Dumbbells and Weights:** Light dumbbells are useful for strength training and can be adapted for various exercises. Adjustable weights or kettlebells can also provide versatility.
- **Stability Balls:** These can be used for balance, core strength, and flexibility exercises. They are also beneficial for low-impact workouts.
- **Chair Yoga Props:** Chairs with sturdy backs, yoga blocks, and straps can support modifications and adaptations for chair yoga.

b. Further Reading

- **"The Arthritis Foundation's Guide to Good Living with Osteoarthritis"** - A comprehensive resource on managing arthritis through exercise and other lifestyle changes.
- **"Osteoporosis: A Guide to Prevention and Treatment"** - Provides information on osteoporosis management, including exercise recommendations.
- **"The Heart Disease Prevention Cookbook"** - Offers insights into heart-healthy eating and exercise practices.
- **"Chair Yoga: Sit, Stretch, and Strengthen Your Way to Better Health"** - A guide to chair yoga practices and modifications for various abilities.
- These resources provide valuable information and support for adapting workouts, staying motivated, and achieving fitness goals.

This newfound unity was not without its hurdles. Eleanor faced opposition from professors stuck in their conventional ways, some refusing to change, others dismissing their efforts as fanciful. But with every challenge, Eleanor remained undeterred. She knew that the path towards understanding had always been paved with resistance.

Orion, too, faced his share of trials. Not all of the supernatural beings were keen on revealing their existence to humans, viewing it as a risk to their long-preserved secrecy. Yet, Orion reminded them that hiding did not equate to peace. He assured them that this wasn't about exposure, but about creating a safer environment for all—the supernatural beings included.

As they navigated these challenges, Orion and Eleanor found solace and friendship in each other. They had begun this journey as strangers, separated by their differing experiences, yet destiny had intertwined their paths. Now, they stood together as partners, their strength and resolve fanned by the collective trust they had braved against the storm they had faced together.

Perhaps the most significant testament to this new era was the change in the atmosphere around Nightfall. Where once rumors and whispers of the supernatural caused fear and distrust, they were now met with curiosity, followed by understanding. The students, once divided, were now united under the shared banner of knowledge and coexistence.

As the ultimate symbol of their success, at the end of the academic year, a grand festival was held: "The Harmony Festival". This event celebrated the unity and the peace between the human and supernatural worlds, becoming a tradition that would be carried forward to mark the dawn of a new era in Nightfall University.

And so, under the moonlit sky and against the backdrop of laughter and cheer, Orion and Eleanor stood together, their hearts swelling with satisfaction and hope. They had ignited a change that would illuminate many generations to come, a beacon of peace and acceptance in a world once towering with division. Their legacy was just beginning...

The end